Law of Attraction Guide

Learn Visualization, Manifestation Techniques and Positive Affirmations, Conceptualize your Goals and Success, Improve Self-Confidence and Reduce Negative Thoughts

Table of Contents

Introduction

All human beings, both large and small, would love to make their dreams come true. But in reality, only a small percentage of humans actually live out their dream, while the rest are dispatched into the pit of failure. When someone fails to realize their dream, they obviously feel bad about it, and even though some people console themselves and give it another shot, most people throw their hands up and cry defeat. Success is guarded by a set of laws. These laws, or principles, must be applied in order to achieve success. The people who achieve success have simply incorporated most of these principles into their lives. They may have encountered failure as they tried to figure out their way, but they never gave up, but instead kept trying until they had knocked on success's door. This book aims to lay bare these laws of attraction so that the reader may understand what it takes to achieve success. The reader will finally understand how to court success.

Part One: Principles of Laws of Attraction

Chapter 1: Intense Desire

Setting goals is one thing, but having those goals come to life is a different matter altogether. The laws of attraction are centered on the idea that if you grew into a certain mindset and arranged your life in a certain manner, then you'd attract success. The laws of attraction are basically principles that one must abide to in order to attract success in their life. One of the most basic principles is having an intense desire. It is the act of being determined to accomplish a goal; it is considered as one of the most important ingredients for success. You may not have the skills or the mentorship necessary for achieving a certain goal, but when you have burning desire, you can still succeed in making your dreams come true. This explains why inventors such as Steve Jobs and Henry Ford, people who lacked technical training, went ahead to create products that changed the world, and created a lasting legacy for themselves.

Psychologists argue that an intense desire often stems from two areas in life. One of them is being inspired. An individual might be inspired by their role model to follow a certain path in life, which can trigger a burning desire to make their dreams a reality. In this age of advanced technology, people can access information in very many ways, thus even seemingly disadvantaged people can reach out to their idols through a variety of digital media.

Another thing that plants a strong desire for success is the psychological distress of being perceived as a failure, or a weakling. It is a powerful force that triggers people to become hungry for success. For instance, if someone had been considered weak and pathetic during their childhood, it may have hatched feelings of bitterness and insecurity, birthing their hunger for recognition. Such people imagine – and rightly so – that making something of their life may redeem their image and make them worthy of love. Thus, they have an unstoppable drive to achieve their important life goals.

Whether your hunger for success stems from your hardships or whether you are inspired to change your life, understand that having a burning desire for success is one of the most critical elements for making your dreams come true.

Some people would like to achieve their goals but they somehow lack an intense desire to keep them persistent. This question comes up, "Can desire be activated within a person?" And the simple answer is "Yes!"

The following tips will help you develop a burning desire to achieve your important life goals:

1. Burn the boats

In this situation, you make the conscious decision of pushing yourself beyond your limits. For instance, if you spot a market gap in the tech scene and you have a brilliant idea on how to capitalize on that opportunity, you may not be acting as aggressively as you ought to, and this could water down the potency of the idea. In such a situation, you might consider putting yourself in the proverbial "do or die" situation. Thus, you may have to get rid of things that slow you down from being aggressive. For instance, you may hand in your resignation letter, and without a job you are in a desperate situation, which will kick in your survival instincts and force you to start pursuing your dreams aggressively.

In Sun Tzu's masterpiece, *The Art of War*, he teaches that soldiers will fight most viciously when they don't have a second option. In ancient eras, it was not uncommon to see an army invade an island, and their general would command that they destroy all the ships, so that they either conquered their enemies or perished. This attitude caused the soldiers to be particularly ferocious.

The cold hard truth is that anything worth achieving never came easy. If you are not "hungry" enough, you are likely to become humbled by obstacles. But when you pile pressure on yourself, you will be in a position to fight ruthlessly.

2. Enhance your environment

Another method of heightening your hunger for success is through enhancing your environment. You achieve this by surrounding yourself with things that remind you of your end goal. Augmenting your environment augments one of the most important factors for success: the subconscious mind. You achieve this by stationing symbols of the success that you intend to replicate at designated places. For instance, if you intend to create a multimillion-dollar company, you may put images of your model company around your office, this allows you subconscious to absorb the idea that you are aiming for the skies. When you are working toward a goal, it is extremely important that your subconscious mind believes you can achieve that goal, or else it might sabotage your efforts. You may even ape the style of your idol. Spice up your office and your company by infusing the management styles of your idol into your life. These seemingly simple influences can boost your drive.

3. Surround yourself with the right people

There's no shortage of negativity in the world. In fact, negativity will always come looking for you, and it is up to you to shun it. You should network with people whom you share similar ideals with, and above all, people who have a positive mindset. Negativity operates like a virus. You can be affected for as long as you are close to a person that holds it. But when you spend time with people that you share values with, they will not only encourage you to keep going, but they'll also become your inspiration and open your eyes to the goldmines of opportunities within your reach. Only disclose your life to those who have demonstrated that they care about you.

Be extremely selective about whom you spend time with. You cannot be an angel and keep the company of demons, and in this case, demons are the people whose way of living contrasts your values. When you associate with a person, you end up picking up their traits slowly, and vice versa.

When you find out that you are spending most of your time with the wrong crowd, it can be a bit hard to escape them, but you should spare no effort in pulling yourself away. The aftermath can be ugly when feelings are triggered, but in the end, it will be the best decision you ever did. Understand that success is reserved for the strong. So, you have to have a warrior mindset in order to create the life that you have always wanted to.

4. Watch what you feed your mind

One of the greatest determinants of success is the quality of information in your possession. You cannot guess your way into success. You have to have a solid plan. This comes from having quality knowledge. In the modern era, we are blessed to have the Internet, which is a resource that contains vast amounts of data. You can access virtually any type of information via the Internet. In the same breath, there's an overabundance of negative information, and if you are not careful you might end up dumbing yourself down. Books are one of the best resources that anyone could ever access. By reading books, you acquire critical data, and also entertain yourself. Thanks to the Internet, books are no longer expensive, as you can download an electronic copy at a much low price than the hard copy (but if you have sufficient disposable income, by all means buy hard copies). When you look at nearly everyone who has done extremely well, you will realize that they have one thing in common, and that is the fact that they are into books. Great books shape how you think and they help you make the best use of your resources. Just as it is important to acquire helpful information, it is also necessary to stay away from negative information. There's an incredible amount of negative media out there. They employ clever marketing gimmicks to hook you. But you must recognize them for what they are: a scam. One of the types of negative media you ought to stay away from is pornography. Studies show that porn has a negative effect on the functioning of the brain.

5. Strategize and put a time limit to your goal

Your desire for a particular outcome is not meant to last forever. You must utilize it when it is still potent. As time passes, new concerns and challenges will take your first priority. So, learn to act when the drive is still there. Draw a plan and implement it. But you must also come up with a time scale for your goal. When you realize that you must fulfill a particular goal within a certain period of time, it will boost your desire.

6. Dressing appropriately

Even psychologists emphasize the need to dress the part in order to attract success. Looks matter. Considering that you will be interacting with other people in order to push your ideas forward, your style ought to elicit a positive reaction. When other people appear impressed by you, and go out of their way to help you, it deepens your hunger for success, as you believe you owe them that.

Chapter 2: Imagination & Conceptualization

Imagination plays a big role in the attraction of success. Imagination implies creativity, and creativity is always in demand. The famous physicist, Albert Einstein, was of the opinion that imagination bears more weight than knowledge, for knowledge has limits, but imagination encompasses the world.

No matter what field you are in, or what role you are playing, there will always be a room for stretching your imagination. If you are not endowed with an imaginative mind, you can still undertake various measures in order to increase your imaginative powers.

If you have a particularly imaginative mind, both your ideas and creations will seem much better than those of your peers. People appreciate creativity. So, when you come out with a wide-appealing idea or product, you make a name for yourself, and get into a position of crafting your perfect life.

The following tips are aimed at helping you boost your imaginative capacity.

1. Open your mind to new lines of thinking

When an idea comes along, most people will jump on it, causing the idea to lose its appeal. Of course it's hard to achieve progress when you're riding on regurgitated ideas. In order to prosper and not merely survive, you must be naturally creative. One of the secrets of achieving this state is adopting an entirely new style of thinking. Instead of sitting around waiting for inspiration, you may venture into the non-mainstream territories and seek new experiences; that's how you gain uncommon insight and expand your creative drive. The greatest thing about imagination is the freedom. You can shape your thoughts however you wish. Thus, you are free to experiment. Once you have experimented enough you may now put together an idea or a product and hope that people will be drawn. Your ideas or products will not always be perfect, and it's totally okay. Once you come up with an idea, never allow yourself to get bogged down by the details. Push it to the world as early as you can. For instance, if you are a software developer, and you intend to make your company an industry leader, you ought to sidestep current trends and start innovating. It is upon you to go the extra mile and come up with something sophisticated. The only downside to being ambitious is the criticism you attract from jealous parties.

2. Dig up knowledge from books

Experience is the best teacherut then it is not possible to perform all the mistakes so that you may learn from them. Books offer a window into reality against varied contexts, and more importantly, they entertain. Books help you prepare for the challenges ahead. No matter what your industry, there'll always be books written by pioneers that will become a guiding light. Success is triggered by your capacity to make the best use of your resources. You need to read more books in order to acquire knowledge and expand your imagination. In this age of the Internet, you have access to a lot of resources, and the distractions are just as much. So, you have to heighten your focus.

3. Tell stories

Two people might tell a similar story before an audience and rouse different reactions. In order to be a good storyteller, you must be quite imaginative. An imaginative person uses words and nuances that paint vivid pictures on people's minds. Telling stories not only increases your imagination but it also strengthens your leadership skills. In order to be termed an effective leader, you must be good at communicating. If Martin Luther King had a meek voice, or stuttered through his speech, he may not have inspired change in America. The ability to communicate is embedded in a person's genetics. It's merely a skill. And anyone can master this skill as long as they are dedicated.

4. Be curious

Another technique of expanding your imagination is through curiosity. The more curious you are, the more your mind will come up with new lines of thought. But in order to be a curious person, you have to step out of your comfort zone, and experience life. You have to bring along a spirit of wonder. When you savor new experiences, your mind naturally raises questions, and this is what drives a person's imagination. Curiosity not only expands your imagination but it deepens your insight into the self. You can learn a great deal about yourself by examining the things that stir your curiosity.

5. Know your passion

It goes without saying that an individual is more proactive over a matter that they are passionate about. One of the reasons that people have a cavalier attitude toward their life is simply because they are doing something that they are not passionate about. But once you discover an idea or a line of work that you are passionate about, your creative drive is resuscitated. Fortunate people discover their passion when they are quite young, and the not-so-fortunate might take decades, or even miss out. Some people ask, "How do I know I have found my passion?" It's simple, that activity will stir up powerful emotions within you.

6. Improve your skill set

You can increase your imagination by diversifying your skill set. With every skill you acquire, you have an opportunity to stretch your imagination. Depending on the skill, you can acquire it either free or by paying for it. The Internet is a great resource for acquiring new skills. To an extent, imagination is really about connecting dots. Thus, for a person who has amassed an impressive set of skills, it becomes easier to connect the dots and come up with a superior idea.

7. Interact with other creative people

There's power in synergy. And that's why it's necessary for creative people to come together. Everyone has a way of thinking that is unique to them, and once people come together, their energies merge together to create something powerful. Thus, push yourself into making friends, and spending time, with your ideological kindred. You may be inspired by their way of thinking and the vice versa is true. Thanks to the Internet, you can establish networks even with people who are oceans away. This improves the diversity and quality of your associations.

8. Learn to have a different perspective

We tend to run low on energy when we consistently hit the wall. But when we are in such situations, we should look for alternative perspectives, rather than giving up. All you have to do is take a hard look. New perspectives help renew our imaginative powers.

9. Practice meditation

The practical benefits of meditation cannot be gainsaid. Meditation is basically an attempt to silence the noise of your mind. This noise emanates from the stresses of living and it manifests as negative energy. Meditation allows us to free ourselves of this negative energy and live with a positive mindset. By getting rid of the negativity, we are in a position to tap into our creative juices, and expand our imagination. The greatest advantage of meditation is that you don't have to pay for it. All you need is a serene environment and some time off your schedule. You will find that by clearing your mind off of the negative energy you can improve your imagination.

10.   Schedule time for imagination

In order to succeed in a particular discipline, you must invest your time, and when it comes to imagination, the same principle applies. Some people only tap into their imagination when confronted by challenges, but ideally, an individual should be exercising their imaginative powers as often as they can. Just as the body requires constant nourishment, your imaginative side requires constant expansion too. You can achieve this by setting aside a particular moment for improving your imagination.

The importance of conceptualization

An idea is born thanks to imagination, but in order to turn an idea into reality, conceptualization is vital. To conceptualize an idea is to basically break it down. It highlights the utility and competitive advantage of an implemented idea. This step is essential as it helps people draw a plan as to how to execute their ideas. The success of an idea is very much dependent on its viability as it is dependent on its ingenuity. It is not enough to access your imagination and discover an extremely forward idea. It also matters that the idea can be implemented in the context of present conditions.

Chapter 3: Positive Affirmation

Positive affirmation is the act of reinforcing a particular belief into your subconscious. This method has been shown to be effective on many times. It helps an individual develop a strong belief that they can achieve their goal.

For instance, if you intend to win an elective seat in your firm, you can recite certain statements over and over in order to cement the idea that you are a winner into your subconscious.

Most of the times we sabotage ourselves because we seem to think that we are undeserving of success and such an attitude obviously keeps us from making use of our full potential.

Most of us are held hostage to negative thoughts that have always distorted reality and caused us to be insecure. One of the biggest triggers of negative thought pattern is abuse. If a person survived abuse, particularly in their childhood, they are likely to struggle with negativity in their adult life.

Affirmations are an excellent way of overcoming negative thought patterns and making your dreams come true. You have to come up with statements that you must repeat over and over in order to align your subconscious mind with your goal.

The following are some traits of positive affirmations:

- They can only influence your behaviors and attitudes: some people try to influence the thoughts and actions of other people through positive affirmation, but they end up hitting a wall. When it comes to positive affirmations, you can only control your actions and thoughts. Thus, the statements should be guided toward yourself. But even though you cannot change someone's mind or actions, you can change your response toward them.
- They should be simple: affirmations should be simple statements with descriptive words. Some people might have a hard time repeating a phrase over and over again if it appears "hard". But crafting a simple statement ensures that you won't have a hard time saying the statement.
- They must be positive: it is vital to have a positive outlook as opposed to a negative outlook. For instance, if you want to advance in your career, you may have a positive affirmation like, "I have won the interview" instead of, "I have not been passed over in the interview". Ensure that your affirmations have a positive connotation.
- In the present tense: affirmations ought to be in the present tense. This elevates your mood and helps your subconscious work toward making your dream come

true. Thus, you should say, "I have the job," instead of, "I will get the job".

o   They ought to be full of emotions: your subconscious mind is particularly receptive to messages that are emotion-laden. Thus, you must ensure that your statements have some emotional weight. In order to achieve this, you have to select your words and phrases a bit more carefully. By tapping into your emotional side, you will be motivated to accomplish your goals.

In order to reap the rewards of affirmation, you have to repeat them consistently. Most people who fail to succeed with affirmations are just noncommittal. And honestly, saying a positive phrase once every three days won't get you anywhere. But when you repeat affirmations as frequently as you can, you will be in a position to make your dreams come true.

Tips for practicing positive affirmations

1. Accompany a positive statement with a natural image

One can make a positive affirmation in a silent voice, but in order to make it more effective, they ought to accompany it with a natural image. For instance, if you want to attract financial success, it is not enough to merely state your wish; you also have to dream up a natural image that represents abundance, for instance, a starry sky. When you learn how to mix these two aspects you stand a much better chance of accomplishing your goals. In order to come up with appropriate images to accompany your positive affirmations, ensure that you are in a relaxed state.

2. Soak in the energy of your goal

Some people imagine that positive affirmation is merely about repeating a statement without engaging other parts of the mind. They are dead wrong. In order to make the best out of positive affirmations, one has to engage all their senses. And this is achievable only through an active imagination. For instance, if you are looking for a job, make a positive affirmation then use your mind's eye to see yourself having that job. Assuming that you want to work for a media house as a journalist, paint an image of yourself with a microphone, reporting on the ground. Living out the experience of a journalist in your mind will speed up the manifestation of your goal.

3. Write an affirmation letter

You might find that your mind wanders off when you try to focus on a goal. You can mitigate this scenario by writing an affirmation letter. In this letter you have the opportunity to outline various things and precisely what you want out of life. Some of the letters you can write include:

- o Write a letter to the universe outlining the things that you want to manifest in your life and how you aim to improve the world.
- o Write down the things that make your ideal day from morning till sunrise.
- o When you fail to achieve a goal, write yourself a letter pointing out the factors that have hindered you from achieving your goals.
- o Write a letter to someone that you hold in high esteem explaining the qualities about them you admire and wish to gain yourself.

4. Utilize your creativity

You can actually infuse your creative juices into your positive affirmations and hasten the manifestation of your important life goals. For instance, you can come up with images, drawings, and music that will add energy into your positive affirmations. For instance, you can put up an image of your goal on the wall, so that every time you look up, it will reinforce your positive affirmations and bring you closer to your goals. You may also compose soothing music with lyrics that speak to your dreams. Once you put on that music, it will boost the potency of your positive affirmations. You may put the file into your phone and have it play at a small volume throughout the day.

5. Use the power of smiling

Positivity is vital when it comes to affirmations. And the subconscious pays attention to our mannerisms and body language. A scowl indicates negative energy, but a smile indicates positive energy. Thus, putting on a smile will boost the energy of our positive affirmations, and accelerate the achievement of our goals. Smiling not only improves our mental status but also invites cooperation from other human beings. When you are struggling with a particularly negative mindset, smiling will help clear negativity, and get started on a positive mindset.

6. Enhance your environment

Recognize that positive affirmation is to an extent a spiritual exercise. You need a ton of peace and tranquility to realize maximum rewards. Can positive affirmations be practiced in a chaotic area? Of course yes. But you will get better results when you practice positive affirmations in a calm area filled with elements of the natural world. Thus, you may do well embellishing your environment. For instance, eliminate the clutter, reduce machine-noise, put flower vases at the corners, and enhance the natural light falling into your room/office. When you have a serene environment, it will boost the potency of your spiritual exercise.

7. Utilize the natural world

Nature emits high-frequency vibrations, and without question, it is one of the best environments to practice positive affirmations. If time allows, you can visit an area rich with natural elements, and soak in the splendor of nature. Take a walk through the narrow paths of a jungle as the trees tower above you and then start your positive affirmation exercise. Considering the reality of modern existence, being surrounded by nature is not in the cards for everyone, but you can purpose to do that when your schedule allows.

8. Meditate

Meditation is the act of calming the noises of your mind. We are commonly surrounded by so much activity, and it seeds unwanted energies in our minds. Meditation is the art of restoring our minds into a state of calm and peace. We achieve this through moving to a quiet area and focusing on positive thoughts while we get rid of our negative thoughts. Thus, when you combine meditation and positive affirmation, you accelerate the manifestation of your goals.

Chapter 4: Focus and Confidence

Focus is the ability to give a task your undivided attention. Most people find it somewhat hard to focus on what they want and it holds them back from living the life that they want. Confidence is the skill of believing in your capabilities. If you don't trust yourself then the world won't either. Most people suffer from a lack of confidence too and it keeps them from utilizing their potential. The following are some tips and techniques for building both focus and confidence:

1. Get quality sleep

Understand that a human being isn't a machine. If you sleep for a mere two hours, or go without sleep, you will be straining your mind, and you won't be productive during the day. On the contrary, if you get sufficient sleep during the night, then you will have much more energy during the day. In order to get quality sleep, you first have to prepare your sleeping environment. Get rid of the clutter, switch off the gadgets, and invest in appropriate lighting. By getting quality sleep, you will have the energy required to carry out the day without a glitch. Your work will seem pretty much easy. On the other hand, if you are low on sleep, you are likely to be exhausted, and you will face your day with lethargy.

2. Get rid of distractions

Another smart way of increasing your focus is by deliberately cutting off "distraction paths". In order to perform with full focus, you have to enter the "zone". This is where you are filled with both inspiration and energy. And your work tends to be of high quality. It is easy to be thrown out of that state by distractions. They come in the form of social media alerts, text messages, voicemail, and TV. Thus, it is critical to shut down these potential avenues of distraction. Turn off your phone and TV, close your door and ensure that any potential distraction has been blocked. This ensures that you can focus on the task at hand and deliver great results.

3. Work in phases

Depending on our age and mental health, we can only go for so long with the same task. We ought to learn in short spans. Generally, the mind tends to wander off after concentrating on the same task for more than a few hours. Thus, it is necessary to take note of when your mind wanders off, and distract yourself with another task. When you regain the focus you can always go back to your important task. For instance, if you are working on a document, you will notice that after two hours of focusing on the document, your mind will start to wander off into other things, and you may have to close your files, perform a mindfulness meditation, and then continue with your work. Studies show that by working while you take small breaks you achieve far more as opposed to working in a long stretch.

4. Improve your diet

You can hardly focus on a task on an empty stomach. But in order to optimize your energy, ensure that you consume appropriate foods. These are foods that are rich in vitamins and vital minerals. By having a balanced diet you are in a position to supply your brain with all the vital nutrients, thus boosting your productivity. On the other hand, if you are not consuming the right foods or worse if you are not consuming enough food, your body will be low on energy, and it will keep you from focusing. Lean meats, fruits, and vegetables, are some of the foods that boost the functioning of the brain.

5. Maintain a work-life balance

At the end of the day, life is not just about work. There ought to be other things that give life meaning apart from our work. These include our, hobbies, spirituality, and most especially, families. You gain the most when you balance out your professional duties with other activities. Some people tend to bury themselves with their professional duties as a way of running away from their "other" life, but such an attitude leads to misery in the long run. You can never run away from whom you are. You ought to face your challenges as it's the only way you can experience growth.

6. Stop comparing yourself to others

Another way that people do a disservice to themselves is by comparing their lives with others. Every person is on their own journey. It's so easy to look at someone who's thriving and consider yourself weak, but you have no idea what that person survived through to get to that point. Learn to stick on your lane and at the same time be inspired to bring out your best. As long as you are improving your life, and not stagnating in mediocrity, you are more successful than you think. When you stick to your business you will always have the confidence to pursue the things that make you a better person.

7. Exercise

The habit of exercising is necessary for increasing both focus and confidence. Exercise relieves your mind of pressure, helps you feel great, and boosts your confidence. When you take to exercise as a habit, you get to improve your looks, and this boosts your confidence. People are superficial and they judge others basing on their looks. Exercise also promotes brain health and increases your focus. It is easy to incorporate an exercising regimen into your life and receive the benefits. You don't even have to invest in a gym membership. There are many freehand exercises you can perform right from your home and improve your looks.

8. Dress sharply

There's some truth to the saying, "You feel good when you look good". Again people judge others by their looks. By investing in a sharp look, you will be sending out the message that you have status, which earns you respect. Always ensure that you are dressed sharply as it will attract people and encourage cooperation. Contrary to what many people think, dressing sharply isn't a costly affair. You only have to make use of your creativity and look for bargains. Before you buy new clothes, spend some time online looking for deals. Also, ensure that you create your personal style. Having your own style helps in terms of improving other people's perception of you.

9. Compliment other people

Almost everyone out there is looking for validation. Thus, a simple compliment wouldn't hurt. You instantly become likable by complementing the people you come across. The apprehension is gone and people become much more open to you. Offering compliments is a nice way of breaking barriers and letting people be comfortable. And once you are comfortable it becomes easier to have a natural conversation.

10.   Get rid of the fear of failure

The fear of failure is a strong force that can hold you back from achieving your dreams. It can also cause you to lose focus and become a weak person. In order to get rid of your fear of failure, understand one thing: that it's okay to fail. Once you understand that there's no problem with failing, you can get started on making your decisions, and following through with them. Fear of failure affects even our productivity. Once we give in to fear, we are unable to improve our creative efforts, and it also causes us to lose sight of our goal. Thus, in order to boost both our focus and confidence, and create the life that we have always wanted, we must get rid of our fears.

11.   Practice being confident

People say, "Fake it until you make it" but in this situation, the right word is "practice". When you were learning to ride a bicycle, on the first day you must have been terrible, but then days later you became competent. It's the same thing with confidence. You have to have the mindset of progress. Even if you don't feel confident deep within you, still ensure that you act like a confident person, and as time goes you will become confident indeed. In order to appear confident even when you are not, do the following:

- o Project your voice
- o Have great body language
- o Practice active listening
- o Be assertive
- o Have empathy

12.   Set goals for yourself

One of the best ways to challenge yourself is by creating goals for yourself. When you have a goal that you want to accomplish you are aware that the stakes are high and this will see you put in the work in order to achieve your goal. When we fail to set goals for ourselves we tend to lose the motivation and focus to keep striving to fulfill our goals. But you must remember one thing: set goals that you can achieve. They have to be realistic goals, and more importantly, you have to set a time limit to the completion of your goals. When you are working toward a goal, you tend to have laser focus, and you have no choice but to be confident, else your dream will go up in flames.

Chapter 5: Profound Self-Belief

Having an unshakeable self-belief is one of those things that are critical to your success. In many cases, you will run into people who will try to hold you back from achieving what you want. But you must not give those people the satisfaction of winning. Instead, ensure that you stand strong for what you believe in. the world is a tough battleground. Simply being talented or skilled is not enough to bring you success. You must have a fighting spirit. This fighting spirit will help you stay focused until you achieve your goal. Some people are so weak that they give up at the slightest change, running into something else imagining that it will be easier. But they find out that their new reality is not any better.

The world around you will constantly test you to find out if you are weak. This is not to mean that everyone is out to get you, but rather an admission that success is not as easy as one might think. One of the men in history that had an unshakeable self-belief was Abraham Lincoln. He endured many personal tribulations that should have made the average man throw hands in the air and cry defeat. But Abraham Lincoln had a goal of becoming president of America. He had an unshakeable belief that he was worthy of leading Americans. So, he kept going at it until he eventually became president.

People who have a strong self-belief weren't necessarily born that way. It's mostly a skill that they acquired along the way. Anyone can develop a profound self-belief and change their lives for the better. You only need to get the right information and start practicing.

The following are some practical tips on boosting your self-belief:

1. See yourself as a winner in your mind

You may be determined to achieve a particular goal, but your negative experiences might be hurting your self-belief, causing you to think that you are unworthy of success. One of the ways to ensure that you always have a strong sense of self-belief is to visualize yourself as a winner. See yourself through your mind's eye that you have achieved what you had aimed for. By acquiring a winner's mindset you will stamp into your mind that you are indeed worthy of success and this will boost your self-belief. Ensure that you practice this exercise on the regular in order to achieve permanent results.

2. Uncover the cause of doubt

One of the reasons why people have such a hard time developing their self-belief is because of doubts. You cannot improve your self-belief without first confronting the root cause of your doubts. Once you doubt your competency, always go back to the drawing board, and look at what may be holding you back from having self-belief. The reasons can be simple or complex. But you have to be honest with yourself. For instance, if you have been married to a narcissistic individual that has always told you that you are incapable of achieving anything, you might want to confront the fact that their criticism affected you. There's no shame in admitting the cause of your doubts. But you also have to take the extra step of getting rid of those doubts so that you remain strong.

3. Silence your inner self-critic

That little voice speaking within you can hold you back from realizing your potential. Suppressing the voice doesn't help matters. The one thing you must do is to provide evidence that contradicts your inner critic. For instance, if that little voice tells you, "You're a loser," you must respond by showing evidence that you are actually a winner. You want to convince your subconscious that you are worthy of success, and when you provide sufficient evidence, then you will increase your self-belief. You may also have to avoid situations that trigger your little voice. In this way, you preserve yourself against negativity.

4. Work on your weaknesses

Don't be one of those people that take excessive pride in their weaknesses. It's not like being weak is something to be celebrated. Learn to work on yourself and boost your resourcefulness. Start by identifying your weaknesses, and then work on these weaknesses, so that you become a better person. For instance, if you realize that you are poor at communicating. Instead of accepting it as a fact of life, you have to start practicing communication skills. As you improve your communication skills you will start to be more confident when you speak with other people, and it will help you develop a solid belief in yourself. Every person has a weakness. But the good thing is that you can overcome your weaknesses if you are willing to put in the work. It is not easy, obviously, but as long as you are persistent, you can work on your weaknesses and become a better person.

5. Motivate yourself

After all has been said and done, you have only yourself to rely on; it is upon you to "save" yourself. Other people may help you, but the drive to go for success must come from you. Thus, you must always motivate yourself for success. One of the ways to motivate yourself is through positive affirmations. These are positive statements that an individual makes in order to rally their subconscious and believe that they are worthy of success. There are very many factors that may put doubts in your mind, but as long as you keep motivating yourself, you are well on your way to developing an unshakeable self-belief.

6. Have a vision

You may be the most skilled, talented individual in the world, but without a vision, you may end up not realizing your full potential. When you have a vision, you channel all of your energy toward its realization, and you are less likely to bow down to pressures. So, sit down and create a vision for your life. Take into account all aspects of your life and ensure that your vision is achievable. This is important not only for yourself but also for those of a similar conviction. For instance, Steve Jobs, the late founder of Apple Inc., was determined to change the world through gadgets, and in the process he inspired millions of people. In the same breath, ensure that you have a vision that can inspire people, and it will give you the energy to stand firm in your beliefs and fight for a better day.

7. Develop your skills

To an extent, your confidence comes down to your competence. If you are good at something, you won't have to shake when dealing with the matter. Also, if you are skilled on a number of fields, you will be pretty confident in your abilities. And confidence is the stepping stone of unshakeable self-belief. Thus, it is extremely important that you develop your skills. In the age of the internet, all the information that anyone could ever need is merely a few taps away, and if it not free, you can still access it for cheap.

8. Keep good company

At the end of the day, we are the average of the people that we spend most of our time with. If we hang out with socially inept, graceless, and cowardly people, we end up becoming like them, and if we go out with positive, confident, and brave people, we end up absorbing their traits. As a person who's determined to develop a firm self-belief, you must keep the company of people that embody your desired trait. This will help you become even stronger in your convictions. There are many activities you can involve yourself to find positive people. Start going out to social events and eventually you will find your tribe.

9. Work on your expectations

Some people, in the name of being ambitious, end up setting too high expectations for themselves, but that's a terrible mindset. If you set unattainable goals for yourself, you will constantly come short of success, and in the long run your subconscious mind will gather enough evidence to believe that you are unworthy of success. In your journey to develop a strong self-belief, you must have your subconscious mind on your side, and you achieve this by ensuring that you are always on winning ways. When you set realistic goals for yourself, you have a much better chance for succeeding, and it will go a long way in boosting your self-belief.

10.   Stay enthusiastic

People who have a profound belief in themselves don't go around with a dead expression. They are lively no matter where they are. It comes down to being a fun person. Keep doing the things you love. And lean towards working with others as opposed to isolating yourself. Having an enthusiastic approach toward life not only strengthens your self-belief but it also boosts your charisma.

Chapter 6: Gratitude

Some of us are not appreciative of the things that we have, and we develop a bad attitude when things don't go our way. This is simply a lack of gratitude. And it can hold us back from experiencing the success that we yearn.

There's nothing complicated about practicing gratitude. It all comes down to the basic attitude of being thankful, both when things are in our favor, or otherwise.

The following are some practical tips on improving our capacity to show gratitude:

1. Keep a gratitude journal

Keeping a gratitude journal helps you take note of the instances that you show gratitude. Ensure that you write down the events that warrant your gratitude. In this way, you will be in a position to appreciate everything that's taking place in your life. Also, note down the less-than-desirable events that you run into and appreciate the lessons that you took.

2. Tell someone that you love them

Not everyone enjoys the warmth of a traditional family, but unless you are very weird, everyone has at least a network of people – a support system – that they rely on. It never hurts to remind these people that you love them. You know love is hard to come by in this world and it is actually nice that you have someone to show you support. Thus, appreciate their efforts.

3. Notice nature's beauty

Some people have a warped sense of beauty. They can only see beauty in shiny and superficial things. You have to deviate from that, and start appreciating the deeper truths of life. The natural world holds the most beauty in life. Thus, ensure that you surround yourself with the natural world, and appreciate the beauty therein. It will help you make nature-conscious decisions moving forward.

4. Nurture your friendships

Friends play an important role in our lives. They lighten the burden and pain that can occasionally come our way. Having great friends is priceless. But then some of us take our friends for granted. This is no good. We ought to learn to appreciate our friends for the incredible role they play in our lives.

5. Smile more often

You may be sad and depressed, but no matter what happens in your life, understand that a better day await you. Thus, put a big smile on your face, and continue living. By smiling often you send out a positive message to the world around you. It makes you endearing. People are drawn to those that radiate love and happiness.

6. Watch inspiring videos

It is important to feed your mind with positive content. Thanks to the internet, you have access to many free videos that could improve your mindset and help you improve your life. Ensure that you are always watching these videos. Also visit websites that talk about positivity. When you feed your mind with positive content, positivity becomes a way of living.

7. Practice kindness on a daily basis

This is a hurting world. There's so much pain around us. And no matter where you are stationed in the world, you just have to stroll outside to see someone who's nursing pain. Thus, you can take it upon yourself to alleviate some of this pain. You can commit to performing an act of kindness at least every day. You don't have to part with millions. It's just helping in a small way. For instance, you can approach an old lady that appears lonely and be there for them.

8. Call your parents much more often

Your parents are the biggest treasure in your life. But as the years go by, your parents get older, and approach their graves. It's a sad reality, but it's the order of the universe. Don't give excuses that you are so busy. A call only takes a few minutes. Ensure that you reach out to your parents every once in a while and find out how they are doing. It will most definitely fill them with joy.

9. Be a volunteer

Another way to show your gratitude is by becoming a volunteer. There are many organizations that are aimed at helping disadvantaged people that you could become a part of. The best way of volunteering is to show up in person and donate your time. But if your schedule doesn't allow that, you can always donate your money and other resources.

10. Stop gossiping other people

If you want to always practice gratitude, you must create an atmosphere of peace around you. One of the ways that people needlessly invite conflict into their lives is by engaging in gossip. So, ensure that you stay away from gossip. It only incites bad blood and antagonizes everyone.

11. Compliment people

Giving someone a compliment won't hurt. Most people appreciate being validated. But this is not to mean that their self-confidence hangs on other people's validation. Thus, when you come across someone that has dressed well, or appears pretty much together, give them a compliment. It will make their day. And that's one more person that you could turn into an ally.

12. Never miss the positive side

When we are tackled by negativity, it's very easy to filter out the good stuff. But we must train ourselves to see the good in bad. For instance, if you are a teenage girl, and you engage in unprotected sex leading to an unplanned pregnancy, it is easy to slide into depression and imagine that your life is over. But you fail to see the bright side of things; that you are going to bring new life into the world; that you are going to nurture and take care of a human being who could end up doing great things for the world. When you find yourself drowning in a sea of negativity, take a fresh look at your circumstances, and realize there might very well be a positive side.

13. Take some time off

There's one person that you must not tire of appreciating: yourself. Don't confuse this mentality with being a narcissist. But you must always be in a position to appreciate yourself for the good job you have done so far. It's really a matter of self-respect. One of the ways to show yourself appreciation is by taking time off your busy schedule to relax and enjoy life. During this moment, you may fix yourself nice meals, lounge at your home, or travel to your favorite destination.

14. Give credit where it's due

Some people, especially people at the managerial level, have a hard time giving credit where it's due. If a company does an excellent job, the manager takes all the credit, never mind that they couldn't care less during the creation phase. Of course that's a deeply flawed attitude toward life. You ought to recognize people for their excellence, especially if they lack power and influence. They don't have to do great things to win your commendation. Small wins are every bit just as worthy of praise.

15.   Be a giver

The reason why many relationships fail is because they tend to be one-sided. This is whereby one party is always giving and the other party is always taking. If you are always taking, understand that you threaten the stability of your relationship, whether it's a personal or business relationship. Learn to be a giver. It shows that you are concerned about the welfare of others. And showing concern endears you to people.

16.   Practice meditation

This is another awesome way of showing gratitude. When you meditate, you are able to tap into the spiritual world, and improve your general characteristics. More people would exhibit great traits if they took up the habit of meditating. The world would be filled with caring people who appreciate the important role that everyone plays in this world.

17.   Stop worrying

Worrying is the one thing that will keep you from living the life that you wanted to. A worrier resents their past, and is fearful of what might happen in the future. And this causes them to become bitter about their lives. Worrying has not even a single advantage. It only hardens your life. Thus, if you'd like to improve your life, to get started on winning ways, you must let go of your worries, and start taking action, since your actions (or lack thereof) play the biggest role in determining your fate.

18.   Practice mindfulness

Mindfulness is all about raising your awareness about the present. It is just about the biggest tip of improving the quality of your life. Stop rushing into things. For instance, if you are dining at a restaurant, avoid swinging your face every which way, looking at the passersby, trying to see who is wearing what, and instead focus on your primary activity: feasting. By channeling all your thoughts into that single activity (eating), you will get to perceive the real taste of your food, its texture against your tongue, and on the whole enjoy your meal. In a sense, you will be appreciating that moment.

19.   Get into the habit of saying "thanks"

It doesn't come naturally to most people. But it is one of the best qualities that an individual could ever have. On many occasions we seek and receive help from other people but fail to say "thank you". And it looks bad on us. When someone lends you a helping hand, the least you could do is appreciate their efforts with a simple, "Thank you". This habit will cause people to want to work with you even another time.

20.   Respect the elderly

You may be on your way to earning millions, possibly billions, through your diligence, but never make the mistake of thinking that you are better than others, particularly your elders. Senior citizens follow kids in being the vulnerable in society. The least you could do for them is show them respect. Showing the elders respect is about doing stuff for them and staying politically correct when you interact with them. Spiritual people believe that doing so would be akin to planting a good karma, and when time is right, you will reap your reward.

21.   Embrace challenges

Don't be one of those weak people who whine about their challenging life. Instead, be a person that revels in challenges. When you come into a challenging situation, treat it as an opportunity to experience growth. Challenges will always be there for as long as we live. Thus, we must learn to have a positive attitude during challenging periods and take them as an opportunity to get to the next level.

22.   Extend an olive branch to your foes

Our self-serving interests, and our endless pursuit for money, are not more important than peace, laughter and harmony. What use is success if you have no one by your side to share with? So many people spend their youth being ruthless masterminds, alienating everyone in their lives, only to end up with a lot of money in their old age, but no one to share the money with. It's the most painful feeling in the world. Thus, learn to extend an olive branch to your foes. If someone is your sworn enemy, be bold and try for peace. As much as it is important to take care of your present interests, don't neglect the future.

23.   Offer your knowledge

This is actually better than dishing out cash. Think about it. If you are an authority on a subject, you can share your knowledge with others, and they will use your tips to replicate your success, or even achieve more than you did. You can purchase a domain and webhosting and set up a website for sharing with the world your truths. This is a massive way of appreciating everyone. As a successful person, you ought to prioritize mentoring people, recruiting your own army of believers; so that when you depart the earth (of course you won't live forever) there'll be a legacy behind you.

Chapter 7: Habits of successful people

There's no sweeter feeling than making your dreams come true. We call it success. But success is rare. Not many people have tasted of success. Of course anyone can apply the appropriate measures and realize success, but then not everyone is aware of these techniques, and for those who are aware of them, not all follow through with the implementation. Success is a massive deal, but in order to taste of it, you must take massive action. The following are some of the habits that all successful people share:

1. They are persistent

This is the ability to keep going despite falling many times over. The successful person is like a soldier trudging along the desert with enemy arrows landing on their back, and although the arrows are painful, they won't overwhelm the soldier to cause them to sprawl on the ground and cry defeat. They hang on to the end. When you first try for success, you will encounter frustration from many corners. People won't be enthusiastic about your plans. Your propositions, offers, suggestions will be turned down. You will even get disrespected. And the thought of giving up will fill up your mind. But you must show persistence, you must keep on trudging along these desert lands until you arrive at an oasis.

2. They have realistic expectations

Successful people have a realistic idea of what they are capable of achieving. What good is it holding on to a fantasy, telling yourself that you are better than you indeed are, only to come up short? Another term for unrealistic expectations is delusions. They lead to failure and disappointment, and your subconscious mind picks up on these failures, planting a belief within you that you are unworthy of success. Thus, if you want to court success, ensure that you are grounded in reality, as it will reflect in your expectations for yourself.

3. They make good use of their time

Time is the most important resource on earth. You can never multiply time. And successful people are well aware of this fact, so they never waste their time. On the other hand, you will find that failures are wasting their time on mindless things. For instance, social media, gossip sites, and porn, and we are talking spending an entire day on these sites. Understand that in order to achieve success you must be productive, which means you have to make good use of your time.

4. They know how to handle failure

All successful people are failures who never quit. Ask any successful person and they will tell you of the failure – many failures – that they endured. Thus, they have learned how to handle failure with decorum. They understand that the world is watching them, and they cannot afford to handle failure poorly, as it would cost them their reputation. If you are just an average Jack or Jill trying to find your way to success, expect failure to rear its ugly head, and that will be a test of your character. Ensure that you take failure with grace. It not only bestows you wisdom but it also builds up your character.

5. They value teamwork

It takes teamwork to accomplish anything worthwhile. Successful people understand that two is better than one. Thus, they are always looking for opportunities to collaborate with others, so that they can pool together their talents and come up with something major. Working as a team puts you galaxies ahead of a solo-worker. Some people deny that they don't need a team in order to thrive and they end up frustrated by the bulk of the work that they must do, and they usually end up failing. Thus, stop giving excuses that you are not good at mixing with others, and work on your social skills. It will help you become a team player.

6. They have good communication skills

Successful people have mastered the art of communication. They are well aware of the fact that infusing confidence and a little showmanship into your communication not only commands people attention and respect, but it also makes you endearing. Success cannot be had in a vacuum. You will need the cooperation of other people in order to achieve your goals. Thus, it is essential to have sharp communication skills.

Part Two: Important Tips

Chapter 8: Eliminate Negative Thoughts

It may be triggered by a feeling, a memory, or statements made by someone else, but once a negative thought has been sown, it compounds at an alarming rate, and soon you are drowning in a sea of negativity. Whether you have negativity inside of you, or you are surrounded by it, in both cases the toxicity leaks into your life and holds you back from success.

If you aim to scale the heights of success, you must be ready to fight away negative thoughts. The following are some tips on managing and ultimately getting rid of negative thoughts.

1. Try to look at the positive side

When you run into a situation that elicits negative thoughts, you might easily get bogged down by the negativity. But never allow yourself to sink to such lows. Instead, you must look at the brighter side. And no matter how bleak the situation appears, there is always a positive thing about it. You just have to look harder. The following are some of the questions you will have to ask yourself:

- o What's the lesson here?
- o What's the good side to this situation?

o   What can I do differently next time for a better outcome?

By focusing on the positive side of the matter, you get to own the narrative as opposed to reducing yourself into a victim, and you also get to mitigate the damage.

2. People don't care much about your actions or words

Negativity catches on when people start imagining what others may think of them. But the old hard truth is that people couldn't care less what you are doing with your life. It's all in your mind. Other people are busy making survival decisions, taking responsibility of their kids, spouses, jobs, and battling fears of what the world thinks of them. So, when you come around to the realization that the world doesn't really care about you as much as you think it does, you will be in a position to take full control of your life and eliminate negative thoughts. The funny thing is that just as you are afraid of what the world thinks of you, the person next appears also worried of what the world thinks of them.

3. Question the thought

Sometimes you have to be a little philosophical in order to win against negative thoughts. In most cases, a negative thought first sneaks up on you and then balloons into a giant cloud of negativity dripping out every pore of your life. But if you are an introspective person, you can question the validity of the thought. Start by asking yourself whether you should pay attention to the negative thought, and if you answer in the affirmative, what do you stand to gain? When you question a negative thought, you cease being the victim and gain power.

4. Watch what you feed your mind

In this age of technological advancement, negative energy is only a few taps away. Most people spend their time on phones, browsing the internet. We are on social media, seeking some attention, and we are on other sites, consuming all manner of questionable data. If you realize that your negative thoughts stem from your habit of consuming unhealthy media, you have to stop that habit. Of course it is not easy to get rid of a habit that had been so entrenched into your system, but if you are serious about improving your life, then you must stop feeding your mind with negative content, and turn to positive things. Remember, just as there is an overabundance of negative things, there's also too much positive content available on these platforms.

5. Stop exaggerating things

If it won't matter five years from now, then it is not a big enough matter. That's should be your attitude. Thus, when a negative thought pops up, don't blow it out of proportion. Actually, you can take the role of the observer and watch it diminish into irrelevance. But when you notice a negative thought and jump into panic mode, you become susceptible to negativity.

6. Physical exercise

When you notice that negative thoughts have started creeping up on you, just put on your training gear and head to the gym. An intense workout will not only renew your energy but also grant you peace of mind. The negativity will be no more. When you allow yourself to dwell on negativity, you become trapped, and you lose the motivation to fight it off. Sometimes, negativity crops up as a way of your brain to alert you of mental strain, and all it takes to get rid of that feeling is an intense workout.

7. Be kind

One of the best ways of dealing with our negative energy is to spread around kindness. This helps feel better about ourselves and it helps us get rid of that negative feeling. You don't have to do big things in order to be kind to someone. Just an act as simple as buying a homeless person a meal can help you feel better about yourself. And once you feel great about yourself you are in a position to get rid of those negative feelings. Always ensure that you practice kindness; it will not only alleviate negative thoughts, but it will also draw people toward you.

8. List down all the great things about your life

If you are not careful, negativity can cast a dark cloud over all the good things about your life. It makes you blind. But you ought to be smarter than that. Always ensure that you are appreciative of the good things in your life. By showing gratitude you enter the appropriate mindset required to eliminate negativity. Create a list of all the things that are going on well for you. This will actually help you see how greatly you are blessed. And more importantly, it will boost your determination to get rid of negative thoughts, and direct your life into positivity.

9. Take a walk

Sometimes, thoughts can be triggered by our environment, or the people surrounding us. And so it is critical to be vigilant of what or who surrounds us. If you suspect that there's a negative influence around you, then do yourself a favor and pull away. But instead of brooding in a corner, take a walk down a quiet road. This will help get rid of all those negative thoughts.

10. Talk them out

Sometimes we develop negative thoughts because we have suppressed an issue. In such a case, it is hard to get rid of the negative thought, unless we agree to tackle the issue and find a solution. If you have suppressed a certain issue, it is important to find the right person and share with them. It will leave you feeling relieved. However, when you suppress an issue, you will be giving your power away, and it will keep you from enjoying your life. Talking things out with the right people makes people trust you.

11.   Reach out to your friends

Great friends are the perfect support system. Negativity is likely to affect your productivity and bring you down. One of the ways of fighting off negativity is by buddying up with your close friends and engaging in an activity that unites you. When you meet up with your friends and engage in an activity that you enjoy, you will be able to forget about your negativity, and just have fun. Our experiences play a critical role in manufacturing our feelings. Positive experiences lead to positive feelings. Also, you can elect to tell your friends about the negative thoughts, and they may give you tips on how to overcome such a challenge. Never underestimate how much your friends understand you.

12.   Stop having extremely high expectations

We don't acknowledge it, but most of us have unrealistic expectations about ourselves and the course that our life ought to take. What normally happens when things don't go as we expected is that we develop a negative mindset. At this point we may start to think that the world is out to get us and that people are no good. In the long run, having extremely high expectations stops us from living an authentic life. Unless we get rid of these expectations, we are unlikely to overcome negativity.

13.   Address the root cause

Sometimes negativity stems from issues that are not immediately apparent. Some of these issues might go back to childhood or a past terrible event that scarred you. Take a moment to reflect on your life and find out what precisely might be triggering the pattern of negative thoughts. Once you identify the root cause of your negative feelings, you may address the issue and find a permanent solution. In this way, you will get rid of negativity and create the life that you had always wanted.

Chapter 9: Manifest Your Destiny

Most people have a goal that they are toiling for, but sadly not every person gets to accomplish their goal. It is not because they are deficient in any way, but rather they employ unhelpful measures when it comes to pursuing success. The following tips are critical when it comes to manifesting your heart's desires.

1. An attitude of gratitude

Most people are unable to accomplish their goals because they have a very cynical approach toward life. They don't have appreciation for anything they have. Also, their attitude becomes nasty when they miss out on something that they had planned to lay their hands on. For instance, if they had gone for a job interview and never qualified, they may become consumed with bitterness and write the director an insult laden letter. Also, when good things happen to them, they are unable to appreciate them, and they take people in their life for granted. Of course such an appreciative person tends to drive people away and they end up devoid of any meaningful personal relationships.

Thus, you must make an effort to be appreciative of what you already have and to keep a positive attitude even when things don't flow as you had expected. A grateful person is endearing. People are drawn to those who appreciate them. And it boosts your chances of success.

2. See yourself living your dreams through your mind's eye

Your mind's eye is a powerful tool of visualizing the future that you want for yourself. It doesn't matter that you are decades away from living out your dream, but you can still enjoy that experience at the mental level. All you have to do is tap into the power of visualization. Every day sit at your favorite corner and call to mind images of yourself thriving as you hope to in your coming years. Make the images as vivid as possible. But you must also take action in order to make these dreams a reality. It is also important that you are realistic about what you are visualizing. For instance, if you are a toothless, lumpy, obese woman, you have no business imagining yourself as a runway model. While the thought of that is incredibly charming, reality is another story altogether. In order visualization to work, you must be aware of your limits.

3. Create a fitting identity

Start preparing yourself for the success that awaits you by creating a fitting identity. For instance, if you hope to become a hotshot lawyer in Manhattan, study how they dress and talk, and start incorporating those aspects in your daily life. By creating the right identity you will be hinting at your mind that this is what you want to become and it will accelerate the manifestation of your dreams. The importance of creating a fitting identity serves two purposes: boosting self-belief, and creating a public persona. Always remember that you cannot achieve success in a vacuum; that you will always need the support of other human beings, and it is necessary to position yourself fittingly, and have a good reputation.

4. Get rid of the clutter

Appreciate the fact that you are in a continuous state of evolution. Your old self may not be in alignment with your new self or the person that you hope to be. Learn to shed off your old ways and embrace new beginnings. This is very critical for your personal growth. You must also de-clutter your living environment. There are many things that we cling to even though they don't serve any purpose, things that hold negative energy, and we still keep all these things in our living spaces. Of course they are a major psychological hindrance, and it would do us a world of good getting rid of them.

5. Prepare for your dreams

Everyone gets their lucky break, but the problem is that some people are never prepared for it. You don't want to be that person. If you have faith that your desires will manifest, take the necessary measures, to ensure that success won't catch you unawares. For instance, if you have been hoping to attract new clients in your store, acquire new inventory. If you have been hoping to get a new job, then ensure that you buy all the items that your job requires. When your desire comes to fruition, you will have a massive head start, and it will help you create the life that you have always wanted to.

6. Seek spiritual nourishment

Spiritual health is just as important in these matters. Thus, ensure that you take exercises that strengthen your spirit. One of these exercises is obviously meditation. This is an exercise of eliminating all the unwanted energies in your mind and embracing positivity in your life. Regular meditation will improve your spiritual life and increase the clarity over your life. When you have a high spiritual health, you are in a position to take inspired steps, and achieve even more success. Another important step for improving your spiritual health is to ensure that you are feeding your mind with the right content. So, depart from negative media and only consume positive media.

7. Have an abundance mindset

In as much as you are hoping that a particular desire will manifest, you must not reduce your life into that single thing. In other words, avoid being obsessed by it. To ensure that you won't have obsessions, create an abundance mindset. Don't grind your life to a halt because of one thing. By having an abundance mindset, you are ready to take even more actions, and pursue other goals. This ensures that you continue building yourself up. Life happens at a fast pace and if you slow down you might end up tossed out of the race. Thus, keep many balls in the air, and this way, you will never find yourself having to throw your hands up and cry defeat.

8. Utilize your gut feeling

We have not made sufficient scientific advancement to make sense of the working of intuition, yet we know that it is a powerful force. Everyone has an intuitive side, but the problem is that we have buried it under tons of negative energies. One of the exercises we can perform to restore our intuition is meditation. Thanks to intuition, we can discern situations in a heartbeat. We don't have to spend even a second analyzing the facts. Our intuition can guide us into making the right choices in tight situations. But don't disregard your mind altogether. You have to strike a perfect balance between listening to your rational side and intuiting.

9. Have fun

At the end of the day, the things that make us truly happy are free. You don't have to chalk your happiness to that HR's call that you are waiting. You don't have to chalk your happiness to your approval by members of the opposite sex. Happiness is your choice. Find fun things to do. Get a laugh. It is never that serious. Having fun is a way of getting rid of the unwanted emotions that have been building up within you. Having fun is a way of increasing your energy levels; so that when you go back to work, you are in a mindset of excellence.

10.   Get rid of worry

Nothing good ever came out of worry. But so many people are trapped in a cycle of worry. They are either attached to their past or obsessed with what may happen in the future. But when they are trapped in worry, the present moment escapes them. Ensure that you are neither a prisoner of your past or future. Keep your mind in the present. This will help you stick to what brings you fulfillment.

11.   Journal

This is the art of writing down the various things that are taking place in your life. When you start journaling, you will realize that your days are quite eventful. You must not forget to include significant mental activities too i.e. thoughts, fantasies, and dreams. Get into the habit of recording the various things taking place in your life and you will gain insight into what you are really about.

12.   Celebrate your wins

Get this: there are no small wins. Every milestone that you complete, every goal that you achieve, is a win. Your subconscious mind is always watching to see whether you are succeeding or failing. If you are failing, your self-belief takes a hit, but if you are doing well, your subconscious mind reinforces your self-belief and increases your willpower. So take every win as a chance to prove to your subconscious mind that you are worthy of success.

Chapter 10: Meditation & Self-Affirmation

Your attitude, thoughts, and perception determine what you attract into your life. If you have negative thoughts, obviously you are bound to attract negativity into your life. Under such circumstances, it would be hard to accomplish your important life goals. You have to get rid of negativity and emotional baggage in order to enter a positive state of mind. Meditation is one of the most effective ways of getting rid of unwanted emotions and at the same time developing a positive mindset.

Many successful people have confessed that they are big on meditation because it helps them get rid of negative energy and increase their focus.

The beauty of meditation is that it has no barrier. You don't have to part with money in order to meditate. It's an exercise that can be practiced by anyone.

Benefits of meditation

1. Improved brain health

One of the benefits of meditation is the fact that it boosts brain health. When your brain is functioning at an optimum level, you have a sharp focus, and it helps you advance much quickly. Researchers found out that people who meditate on a regular basis tend to upgrade about nine regions of their brain, which results in the following benefits:

- o Improved cognition
- o Decreased stress
- o Increased happiness
- o Quality sleep
- o Improved learning
- o Improved memory
- o Higher EQ and IQ

2. Defying age

A person who meditates regularly is no stranger to the statement, "You don't look your age!" Meditation helps them look younger than they really are. And then people who meditate tend to live far longer than average people. It's no secret that people are superficial. People judge you by your looks. But then an individual that meditates is likely to be in great shape and also have healthy skin.

3. Weight loss

Some forms of meditation combine spiritual and physical exercise. These combined exercises help an individual burn excess fat and lose weight. Having weight issues poses various health risks and on top of that it can lower an individual's self-image.

4. Strengthens immunity

Meditation improves the building blocks that are responsible for our immune system. The immune system is our body's defense mechanism. When disease agents come knocking, our immune system rises to the occasion, and fights away these agents. Practicing meditation on a daily basis strengthens your immune system and elevates you into a high health status. And it is no secret that health is vital in making progress in life. You have to be in good health to be able to implement your decisions and chase your goals.

5. Lessens anxiety

Anxiety is one of the most common forms of mental illness, with an estimated 40 million adults in America battling the illness every year. The figures could be worse considering that not every American is sensitized about mental illnesses. Meditation has been shown to eliminate symptoms of anxiety. Meditation, unlike commercial pills, promises permanent results, and this is because meditation helps a person tackle the root cause of their mental illness.

6. Willpower

There are so many people out there who have "potential", but sadly they get overwhelmed by reality, and end up dropping out of the race. In a sense, these people lack willpower. The world is a tough battle ground, and it takes someone with a fighting spirit to achieve their goals. Willpower is the act of hanging on even when you should be discouraged, trusting that you have something of worth, and never yielding until you get your way. It is an extremely important skill for survival in the modern world. Willpower goes together with mental stability. Meditation improves an individual's mental health; in that sense, meditation equips an individual with the ability to be persistent in their quest for success.

7. Creativity

No matter what area you can think of, there'll always be a need for creativity. Creativity never goes out of style. The awesome thing is that people are naturally creative, but most of that creative energy has been buried under negative emotions, distractions, and inactivity. People who meditate on the regular tend to have a higher creative energy. This boosts their competency when compared against non-practitioners. Creativity always stands out and it's more often than not rewarded.

8. Intuition

Intuition is the ability to comprehend a certain scenario even without looking at the facts or evidence. It's also called gut feeling. Sometimes, our intuition may contradict our rational mind, and in a world that puts a lot of emphasis on being rational, intuition gets a bad rap. But amazingly, ultra-successful people have confessed to using intuition more than their minds, when making key decisions. Steve Jobs, founder of Apple Inc., once said, "Intuition is more important than intellect". Warren Buffett relies on his intuition when buying out a company. And even Bill Gates uses his intuition to make key decisions. Of course this is no encouragement to use intuition at the expense of your mind. You should strike a perfect balance.

The benefits of meditation are endless. But most people seem to have a misconception about meditation. There are no barriers to practicing meditation. You can perform at any serene environment. Some people think that meditation is a light exercise, and of course they are mistaken. If done the right way, meditation is an extremely taxing exercise, and this is because it consumes a huge amount of mental resources.

A seemingly simple meditation exercise involves the following steps:

Step one: being comfortable

You start off by assuming a comfortable position. You can be sitting, standing, or lying on a bed. You basically assume a position that feels most comfortable. Comfort is necessary as it will allow you to assemble together the focus needed to practice meditation.

Step two: close your eyes

Can you meditate without closing your eyes? Of course, yes. But when you close your eyes you get to raise your concentration and improve the experience. In fact, you can even put on an eye mask to achieve your aim.

Step three: breathe

At this point, you now have to focus on your breath. Let it be natural. As you focus on the inhalation and exhalation process, pay attention also to how other parts of your body respond. Place your hand at different parts of your body and pay attention to how you are feeling. Finally, you may start observing your thoughts. Some of them will be positive and others will be negative. You will have an urge to fight the negative thoughts, but you must not do it. Just take the role of an observer and watch your thoughts pass across your mind.

Types of Meditation

1. Mantra meditation

As the name implies, this type of meditation is about repeating a word or phrase, a *mantra*, in order to achieve a certain goal. The mantra meditation is most effective during periods of emotionally-charged events. For instance, if you are engaging in a competitive sport, and it is the finals, you can practice mantra meditation in order to get into a winning mindset. Also, if you are sorrowful, you can practice mantra meditation in order to overcome the grief and be happy again.

2. Walking meditation

Some people are not into "still meditations". The biggest reason is anxiety. Also, some people have a strenuous schedule, which means they haven't the time to sit still and meditate. Such people have an alternative choice in walking meditation. The walking meditation, as the name implies, is practiced when an individual is walking. As they consciously put one step in front of the other, preferably down a quiet road, they may inhale and exhale carefully, while watching their thoughts. If they are walking down a noisy road, they can plug in earpieces and take a listen to soothing music. Walking meditation combines both spiritual and physical aspects to raise the individual into a higher plane of wellbeing.

3. Mindfulness meditation

In this form of meditation, one is brought back to their present. So many times we are distracted and held back from completing our immediate goal. For instance, if we are at a restaurant having a meal, we might get distracted by other things or people near us. This keeps us from enjoying our meal. Mindfulness meditation is particularly used for restoring your senses to the current moment. In the case above, you start by shutting down your peripheral vision, and turning on your tunnel vision. This is to simply stop watching the world from the corners of your eye and turn your full attention to the food before you. And then next you have to focus on the sensations that the food elicits. Pay attention to the texture of the food against your tongue, the taste, and the aroma. This will allow you to savor your food at a much deeper level.

4. Loving kindness meditation

This type of meditation is practiced in order to boost positive emotions within us or to send them out towards a particular person or thing. This type of meditation is beneficial during hardships, either at a personal level, or about someone you care about. You start by assuming a comfortable position, preferably sitting cross-legged on the floor, and then close your eyes, and start calling to your mind positive energies. If a negative thought crosses your mind, fight it away. Call to your mind feelings of joy, happiness, merry, and also visualize people having fun. Soak in that energy.

Chapter 11: Achieve Goals with the Art of Visualization

Our present reality is a sea of energy. A positive state of being comes with high-frequency vibration and a negative state of being comes with low vibrations. We can engage with the sea of energy around us in order to turn our dreams into reality.

Visualization is a powerful method of courting success. It entails casting out mental energy into the universe in order to make our wishes come true. Through visualization, you create a vivid image in your mind, depicting your end goal. For instance, if you want to grow up into a hotshot lawyer in NYC, you may envision yourself in the office, signing on high net worth clients.

Many successful people have confessed to using this method to achieve their goals. Visualization is one of the primary elements in the laws of attraction. If you follow the guidelines of visualization, you will achieve your goals too.

Visualization is not akin to sending out a wish to the universe. It is actually about living out your dream. You get to see yourself already having what you yearn for.

Visualizing your dreams on a daily basis will see you make your plans a reality much sooner.

Benefits of visualization

The following are some benefits of practicing visualization on a regular basis:

1. It promotes creativity

Thanks to visualization, your brain enters a phase of unparalleled creativity. Visualization has a huge impact on your subconscious mind, triggering a desperate search for a method to make your important goal materialize. When your creativity levels go up, you acquire the resources and the drive to fulfill your important life goals. For instance, if you want to become a best-selling author in three years, you start by visualizing yourself as an award-winning author. While you visualize on the regular, your subconscious mind enters a creative space, fueling your productivity so that you come up with a masterpiece.

2. It promotes brain health

Visualization is a resource-intensive activity that relies on the coordination of various parts of the brain. By visualizing your goals on a daily basis, you get to sharpen your brain, and limit your risk of developing mental illnesses. Other benefits of keeping your mind active include:

- o Improving memory
- o Improving physical health
- o Promoting self-esteem

3. It increases your motivation

Most people want to succeed. But one of the hindrances is their diminished motivation. When you lack sufficient motivation, you are unlikely to take action, and consequently you will be unable to reach your goals. By visualizing your goals, you get to experience, albeit mentally, what it is like to live out your dream, and this can inspire you to take action and make your goals a reality.

The "Mental Rehearsal" Visualization Technique

This visualization technique is mostly used in preparation for victory. Elite athletes have confessed to using this technique to not just win but smash records.

To achieve results, the "mental rehearsal" technique must be practiced consistently, preferably on a daily basis. The best time to practice visualization is a matter of personal preference, but early mornings and bedtime are quite appropriate, as this is when you are most relaxed.

Step one: create the right atmosphere

The first step in practicing "mental rehearsal" visualization is ensuring that you are comfortable. The best position is to sit on a couch in a serene environment facing a mildly bright wall. Next up, you must close your eyes, and call to mind a scene of a movie theater. Take your time to envision all the little details of the movie theater. See yourself in the seat holding onto your popcorns; the dimmed lights; the little body movements, the moviegoers under the dim lights, and other things common in a movie theater. On the monitor, envision the perfect setting for the manifestation of your goal. For instance, if you intend to become a top grossing musician, you can envision a large wild crowd waving and crying out the artists name before they step on stage.

Step two: enter the dream world

Now that you have simulated the environment of a movie theater within your mind, it is time to step into the virtual reality that the moviegoers are watching. Slowly, get up from your seat and walk up to the monitor, and step through into the virtual world, so that you are the much awaited performing artist. Watch the crowds cheer your name as you take center stage and the spotlight falls on you. Now you may start rocking the revelers with hit after hit, dancing on stage like the superstar you are, with the crowd cheering itself hoarse. Now you are living the dream of a top grossing superstar.

Step three: step out

Slowly, bring your gig to a close, turn around and walk away from the stage, stepping through the monitor and back into the movie theater. The moviegoers should still be watching as though everything is normal. On the screen, you should still be up there on stage, dancing and singing as if you never left. You may reach your hand out to point at the monitor, shrinking it into a round mini-player, and then you may pull it toward your mouth and swallow it. By gobbling up that monitor is an action of transmuting that energy so that it will hopefully manifest in real life someday.

Creating Goal Pictures Technique

This form of visualization doesn't use extensive mental resources to perform. It's about putting yourself in an environment that corresponds with your goal. For instance, if you intend to become a movie actress, you can take a poster of a top grossing film and put a cutout of your picture into the poster. Once you put your image in an environment that reflects your goal you may hold the picture against your nose in order to transmute that energy.

Index Cards

Using index cards is a great way of achieving your day-to-day goals. You may practice this kind of visualization at bedtime, preparing for the day ahead. Write down the goals that you aim to complete the following day. And once you are done, go through them, using your imagination to see yourself putting in the necessary work to accomplish your goals, and once you are done looking at your goals, you may hold the index cards against your chest, or put them under your pillow, as you drift to sleep.

Conclusion

The first principle of attracting success is having an intense desire. This is basically having a burning wish for a particular goal. Many successful people have confessed that they got into their line of work because they had an intense desire for it. A burning desire is vital as it keeps you going even when you have reason to be discouraged. Another principle of success is imagination. This is basically an individual's capability to tap into their creative energy and come up with something worthwhile. When you are on the plane of imagination, there are no limits. A big imagination inspires you to be unique and it helps you stand out. One must also be focused, and must have confidence, in order to realize success. Focus is an individual's capacity to eliminate distractions and work on their goal with a single purpose. Confidence is the ability to view oneself as deserving of success and to actually follow through with actions. The book discusses many principles which are essential for success.

Description

Your thoughts, beliefs, attitudes, and habits determine whether or not you will attract success. Although everyone is in pursuit of success, only a small percentage of people manage to achieve what they set out for. And it's not that they are incompetent; it's simply because they haven't put to use the various principles of success. This book outlines the various laws that attract success. The laws are not things you have not heard of, except that there's a science to their application. You have to practice these laws together, not separately, in order to see results. Many successful people have admitted to using these principles to court success and create the life that they had wished for. Some of the topics covered in this book include:

- o Intense desire
- o Profound self-belief
- o Gratitude
- o How to manifest your desires
- o Tips on eliminating negative thoughts
- o Meditation

This book will help the reader improve the quality of their life and start winning.

www.ingramcontent.com/pod-product-compliance
Lightning Source LLC
Chambersburg PA
CBHW020328290526
45785CB00007B/2961